D0436781

YOGA
FOR TODAY

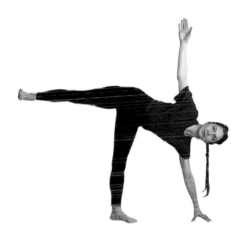

Suzanne Pattinson

Haldane Mason

First published in the UK in 2000 by
Haldane Mason Ltd
59 Chepstow Road
London W2 5BP

Reprinted 2001 (twice)

Box Set – ISBN: 1-902463-19-6
Book – ISBN: 1-902463-60-9

A HALDANE MASON BOOK

Editors: Jean Coppendale, Jillian Stewart, Beck Ward
Design: Louise Millar
Photographer: Sue Ford

Colour reproduction by CK Litho Ltd, UK

Printed in China

Acknowledgements
The publishers would like to thank Ingrid Ballard, Jeffrey Fernandez, Ben Keith
and Suzanne Pattinson for being such willing models, and Suzanne for all her
help on the photo shoot.

IMPORTANT
Yoga should be practised in full awareness of your body: never force
yourself into positions that feel uncomfortable or difficult to get out of.
The information in this book is generally applicable but is not tailored to specific
circumstances or individuals. If in doubt about any of the postures or routines
described, please consult a qualified yoga teacher or doctor.

Contents

The Art of Yoga   4

Warm up to Yoga   8

Stretch with Yoga   16

Relax with Yoga   32

Yoga at Work   40

Yoga and Pregnancy   48

Yoga Programmes   56

Index   64

The Art

OF

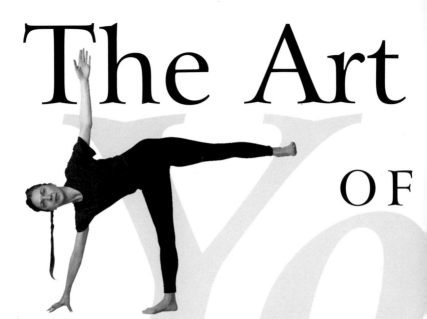

T *he word 'yoga' is an ancient Sanskrit term meaning union.*
Behind the word is a complex set of philosophical systems
and disciplines, deep rooted in Indian history.

The yoga we generally practise in the West today represents only a
small part of the entire philosophy of yoga and is known as Hatha
yoga, or union by body mastery. Made up of two Sanskrit words 'ha'
and 'tha', meaning sun and moon, this union has two main strands –
breath control and physical postures (known in Sanskrit as 'asanas').

Yoga

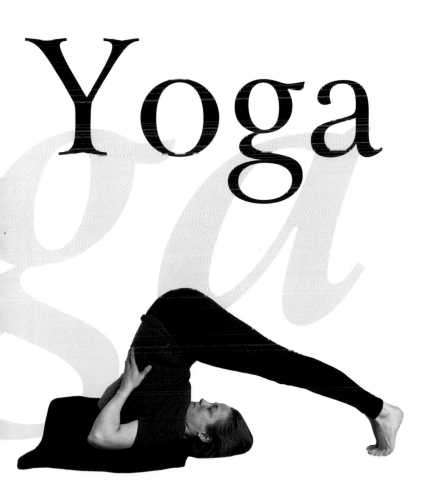

Traditionally regarded as a lower form of yoga, Hatha yoga was practised as preparation for higher forms of yoga involving mental mastery. Today in the West, however, the value of hatha yoga as a method of exercising the body, of making the best use of the breath, and of relieving stress and tension and inducing feelings of relaxation, has promoted it to one of the most enduring and popular forms of exercise and relaxation.

Two principles distinguish hatha yoga from other forms of exercise:
- the postures are synchronized with the breath: the out-breath and in-breath are used to move in and out of postures and, while the posture is held, the mind is focused on the smooth and rhythmic flow of the breath
- the mind is concentrated on the posture: the precise positioning of the body in the postures encourages a quietening of the mind, as well as greater body awareness

Yoga is not just a sport or a form of exercise but is something much richer and more spiritual. Its ability to challenge the body and at the same time to quieten and control the mind brings physical and mental fitness closer together like no other activity.

Yoga does not require any complex equipment, just a few simple 'aids'. A yoga belt is extremely helpful for use with several postures, as is a foam block (this could be replaced with an old telephone directory or a book of a similar size). A non-slip mat is ideal to stand or sit upon, but alternatively practise on an unslippery floor. Any other aids that are required, such as blankets and cushions, can be found around the home. Note that you will need to wear loose clothing with bare feet, and shouldn't practise if you have eaten a heavy meal in the preceding three hours.

This book makes no assumptions about your experience of yoga, your knowledge of the postures or your level of fitness and suppleness. It will suit you if you have been attending yoga classes and now wish to work on your own at home; it will also suit you if you are new to yoga and wish to try out some postures by yourself. The range of postures – together with suggestions on how to make them easier, harder or more restful – is designed to satisfy people of varying abilities.

Many yoga postures do not have English names; each posture is given its Sanskrit name and the English translation in brackets after, where one exists.

The following organizations and people will be able to supply information and equipment on yoga:

In the UK
The British Wheel of Yoga
1 Hamilton Place, Boston Road,
Sleaford, Lincolnshire NG34 7ES
Tel. 44 (0)1529 306851
Fax: 44 (0)1529 303233
www.members.aol.com/wheelyoga

Iyengar Yoga Institute
(Maida Vale), 223a Randolph Avenue,
London W9 1NL
Tel: 44 (0)20 7624 3080
Fax: 44 (0)20 7372 2726
www.iyi.org.uk

Light on Yoga Association (UK)
Tel: 44 (0)1604 714590
www.loya.ukf.net

Ruth White
Church Farm House, Spring Close
Lane, Cheam, Surrey CM3 8PU
Tel: 44 (0)20 8644 0309
www.ruthwhiteyoga.com

In the US
*Iyengar Yoga National Association
of the United States*
Tel: 1 800 889 9642
www.comnet.org/iynaus

The Yoga Site
www.yogasite.com

In India
The World of BKS Iyengar's Yoga
www.bksiyengar.com

In Australia
Iyengar Yoga School of Kuringgai
Roseville, Sydney
Tel/Fax: 61 2 9416 5537
Email: willetts@dot.net.au

Yoga Synergy
PO Box 3017, Waverley, 2024
Tel: 61 2 9389 7399
Fax: 61 2 9389 7238

Western Australian School of Yoga
10 Queen Street, Perth, 6000
Tel/Fax: 61 8 9481 6113

In Canada
Yoga Centre Toronto
2428 Yonge Street, Toronto, Ontario,
Canada, M4P 2H4
Tel: 1 416 482 1333
www.yogagroup.org

Yoga Studio
344 Bloor Street W., Suite 400
Toronto, Ontario, M5S 1W7
Tel: 1 416 923 9366
Fax 1 416 923 1275
www.yogastudio.net/

Warm up
TO Yoga

This section introduces some straightforward warm-up exercises. Before you attempt the yoga postures in the next section you should always warm up with all or a good many of these exercises. As in any sport or form of exercise, the body needs to be prepared for what is to follow.

The exercises are set out in a sequence, starting with the head and moving down the spine to the feet and ankles. They are a mix of simple exercises and basic yoga postures.

The exercises follow some basic yoga principles:
- aligning the body so that both sides are balanced
- working with the breath to move in and out of the posture
- holding the posture for a number of seconds – the exact number is not given but aim for a minimum of about 10 seconds
- relaxing the mind while maintaining body awareness

You should be able to carry out most of these exercises no matter how inexperienced or unsupple you fear you are. Some of the exercises assume a kneeling position. If you find it difficult to kneel, place one or more cushions between your feet and buttocks. In a few instances, modifications are suggested to make the exercises easier.

THE NECK

The neck is prone to stiffness, particularly if you've slept or rested your head in an awkward position. These two exercises increase the blood circulation in this area, stimulate the nerves and increase mobility of the head in all directions.

1 NECK 1

Sitting or standing, hold the head erect, tucking the chin in slightly to stretch the back of the neck. Breathe out and let the head drop. Look down towards the chest and feel the stretch in the back of the neck. Take a few breaths in this position, then breathe in and raise the head.

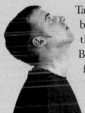

Take a few breaths, then breathe out and drop the head backwards. Breathe normally for a few seconds, keeping the face and the eyes relaxed. Breathe in and raise the head.

Breathe out and turn the head to the right, taking the chin round towards the right shoulder. Breathe normally for a few seconds, then breathe in and return the head to its original position. Repeat on the left side.

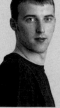

2 NECK 2

Lie on the floor on your stomach and cup your chin in your hands with your elbows bent on the floor in front. Breathe out, let the elbows move forwards and gently push the head backwards. Hold this position, breathing normally, keeping the shoulders down and the face relaxed. Breathe in and pull the elbows towards you, allowing the head to come up.

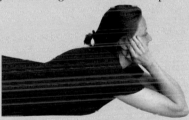

With the elbows pulled under the shoulders, clasp the hands over the crown of the head. Breathe out and pull the chin towards the chest. Hold for a few seconds, breathing normally. Breathe in and raise the head.

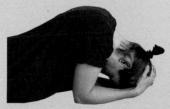

YOGA FOR TODAY

THE SHOULDERS

The shoulders can be a big problem area. It is all too common to see rounded shoulders or badly balanced shoulders, where one is held higher or further forward than the other. These exercises improve posture by encouraging you to broaden the upper chest and flatten the shoulder blades into the back. They also increase mobility in this area.

1 SHOULDERS 1
Parvatasana

Standing with your feet hip-width apart and parallel, interlock your fingers in front of you. Breathe out and stretch your arms forwards and over your head, pushing the palms upwards. Straighten your elbows and push your palms towards the ceiling. Keep the face soft and your shoulders down. Breathe normally and try to take your arms slightly backwards without moving your lower back and hips forwards. Breathe in and lower the arms.

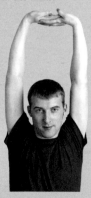

Repeat, interlocking your fingers with the other thumb foremost.

2 SHOULDERS 2
Gomukhasana

Standing or kneeling, bend the left elbow behind your back so that the back of your hand rests high up the spine – between the shoulder blades if possible.

Stretch the right arm up, then bend the elbow and clasp the left hand. Breathing normally, check that your face is relaxed and your head is straight.

Unclasp the hands, breathe out and lower your arms to the side.

Repeat on the other side.

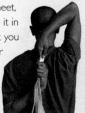

Need something easier?
If your hands do not meet, fold your belt and hold it in the upper hand so that you can clasp it in the other hand. Now work your hands closer together on the belt.

10

THE WRISTS

The wrists tend to be less of problem area than other parts of the body, although they can be aggravated by too much time spent at a keyboard. These exercises stretch the long tendons that run from the forearms into the hands.

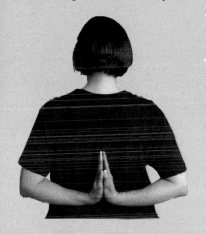

1 WRISTS 1

Standing or kneeling, join the palms behind your back with the fingers pointing upwards. Take the hands as high as possible between the shoulder blades, pushing the palms together. Relax the face and the shoulders, breathe gently and feel the upper chest broaden. To come out of the posture, lower the arms and rest your hands at your sides, turning the palms forwards to relieve any stiffness.

2 WRISTS 2

Kneeling, put your hands flat on the floor in front of you with your fingers facing towards you, thumbs on the outside. Your shoulders should be directly above your wrists.

Breathe out and gently move your body backwards, keeping the heel of your hands flat on the floor. Hold for a few seconds, breathing normally. Breathe in and return your body to its original position.

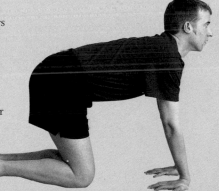

THE BACK

The back is the most important part of our structure and, unfortunately, the most prone to strains, sprains and stresses. It has great potential to flex forwards, backwards and sideways, as well as rotate. Yoga is excellent at stretching and strengthening the muscles in all these directions. These two exercises stretch the back lengthways, while the postures in the next section do the rest.

1 BACK 1
Hastasana

Standing tall, with your feet together, breathe out and stretch the arms forwards and up, palms facing inwards. Breathe normally and stretch the arms up higher, without letting the lower back and hips tilt forwards. Breathe in and lower the arms to the sides.

2 BACK 2

This exercise is also good for the shoulders, as well as the back. You will need a ledge to rest your hands on, such as a windowsill, a chest of drawers or the back of a chair.

Stand with your feet hip-width apart and parallel. Stretch the arms above the head, breathe out and lean forwards, placing your hands on the ledge shoulder-width apart. Your trunk and arms should be horizontal and your legs straight and vertical.

Breathe gently, look down towards the floor and feel your spine lengthen between your neck and waist. To come up, you can either drop your arms and unfold your body to a standing position, or breathe in and raise your arms up from the ledge.

Need something easier?

If you found this difficult, you may have chosen a ledge that was too low for you. Move to a higher surface and try again. The higher the ledge, the less likelihood that the trunk will be horizontal (remember to keep the legs vertical).

THE HIPS

The hips are built to be flexible and balanced. Unfortunately, they rarely remain completely balanced and can lose their movement with wear and tear. These exercises aim to restore this flexibility and balance.

HIPS 1

For this exercise you will need a yoga belt and a ledge to rest your foot on.

Stand with your feet together and at right angles to the ledge. Raise the right leg to the side and place your foot on the ledge. Holding the ends of the belt in your right hand, hook the belt round the foot and use it to stretch your spine upwards.

Breathe normally. Check that your raised foot is in line with your standing foot and that your trunk and head are at a right angle to the ledge. Unhook the belt and lower your foot to the floor. Repeat on the other side.

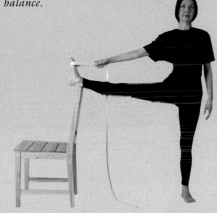

Need something easier?
If you found this difficult, you may have chosen a ledge that was too high. Move to a lower one and try again.

HIPS 2

Find a wall clear of furniture and lie on your back with your knees bent up over your chest. Shuffle in close to the wall so that your buttocks touch the skirting board. Raise your legs and rest them on the wall. Breathe out and open the legs wide, keeping your knees straight. As you breathe out, feel the insides of your thighs release and stretch. To come out, bend your knees over your chest and roll to the side.

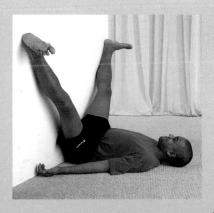

THE KNEES

The knees can be the most vulnerable part of the body, often due to the muscles around them shortening. Always be careful when stretching this area of the body and stop if you feel any sharp pains. The exercises here aim to lengthen the muscles behind the knees.

1 KNEES 1
Adho mukha svanasana
Excellent for the shoulders and back, as well as the knees.

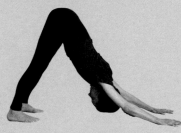

Kneel on the floor and place the hands on the floor in front of you a little wider than shoulder-width apart.

Spread the fingers wide. Lift your knees off the floor and check that your feet are level and about hip-width apart. Breathe out, straighten your legs and lift the hips up as high as you can. You should be balanced on your toes, the balls of the feet and your hands.

Breathe out again and lower your heels towards the floor (if they touch easily, step your feet back). You will feel a stretch in your hamstrings and calf muscles. Relax the head down and feel a strong stretch through your arms, shoulders, trunk and down your legs.

To come down, bend the knees and kneel. Rest your trunk over your knees and lay your arms on the floor in front of you.

2 KNEES 2
You will need a yoga belt for this exercise. Lie on your back with your legs together. Bend your right leg and hook the belt round the underside of the foot, holding the ends of the belt with both hands.

Stretch the leg up, keeping the knee straight. Breathe normally and aim to bring the leg to the point where it forms a right angle with the trunk. (Don't be disappointed if your leg is some way off this point – with practice your hamstrings will soon stretch.)

To come out, unhook your belt and lower your leg with the knee bent. Repeat on the other side.

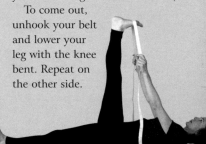

THE FEET AND ANKLES

The feet and ankles work together to support the weight and movement of the body. Flexibility and balance in both helps to maintain balance in the rest of the body. The exercises outlined here help to unstiffen the ankles and stretch the front side of the feet.

1 FEET AND ANKLES 1

Kneel on the floor, placing your feet and ankles close to one another. If you find kneeling uncomfortable, place a cushion between your feet and your buttocks. Sit erect and breathe gently.

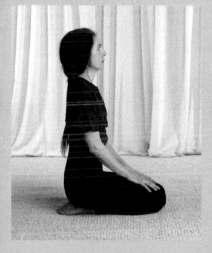

Need something more difficult?
If you can do this easily (without the cushion), use your belt to tie your ankles together. This holds them closer together and gives a strong stretch on the front of the feet and ankles.

2 FEET AND ANKLES 2

Prasarita padottanasana
Also good for the knees and legs.

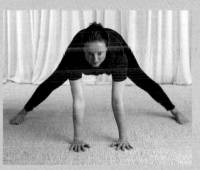

Stand with your legs wide apart (about 1.5 metres or 5 feet) and your feet parallel. Breathe out, lean the trunk forward and place your hands on the floor in front of you. Breathe normally and push the outside of your feet to the floor. Be careful to keep your hips in line with your ankles. Stretch your back between your neck and waist at the same time. To come out, bend your knees slightly, step your feet in a little and lift your trunk up.

Stretch

WITH

This section introduces a mixture of basic and fairly advanced yoga postures. For some of the simpler postures, modifications are suggested to make them more challenging. Conversely, the modifications suggested for some of the more advanced postures make them easier to achieve.

These postures aim to:
- align the body so that it becomes balanced
- stretch parts of the body that are rarely, if ever, stretched in everyday life
- give you a greater sense of body awareness

Yoga

They follow some basic yoga principles:

- working with the breath to move in and out of the posture
- holding the position for a number of seconds – the exact number is up to you as you may find some postures quite tough to hold for long (particularly if you're new to yoga or you're feeling tired)
- focusing the mind on the 'here and now'

Some of the postures shouldn't be attempted under certain circumstances (for example, if you are menstruating). This is indicated in the relevant postures. If you are pregnant, you need to read the section on Yoga and Pregnancy (page 48) before you attempt anything.

Tadasana (THE MOUNTAIN)

This is the basic position from which you will start many of the postures that follow. It may look very simple but it is difficult to align everything perfectly.

Stand with the feet together. Starting with the feet and moving upwards, check the following points:

1 Touch the big toes and inner heels together, stretch out the toes, keeping the feet broad and long.
2 Lift the arches of the feet.
3 Keep the weight of the body even on both feet and balance between the toes and heels.
4 Stretch the legs upwards and keep the knees drawn up.
5 Make sure the lower back is not arched. Tilt the pelvis so that the buttocks are tucked in – in other words, your bottom is not sticking out.
6 Keep the upper chest broad and flatten the shoulder blades into the back (the shoulders will still feel relaxed and wide).
7 Hang the arms and hands naturally at your sides.
8 Keep the back of the neck long, with the chin tucked in slightly.
9 Relax the face and keep the eyes looking straight ahead.
10 Keep the breath even.

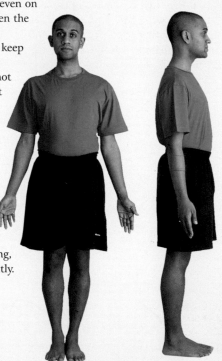

Padmasana (THE LOTUS)

The lotus position is the classic posture for meditation. It is effectively a locked position – once the legs are in position, the lower half of the body has to remain still. Do not attempt this posture if you have problems with your knees. You will need one or two blankets.

1 Take your blanket(s) and make a flat platform.
2 Sit with your legs crossed.
3 Lift up your right leg and with your left hand lift up the flesh of the calf muscle. Place your right foot on the top of the left thigh.
4 Lift your left leg and again lift up the calf flesh with your hand. Raise the left foot over the right knee and place it on the right thigh. Adjust both feet to bring them closer to your hips.
5 Sit erect and place your hands palm up on your knees with your fingers gently curled.
6 You may wish to hold your head erect or lower your chin towards your chest for meditation/concentration.

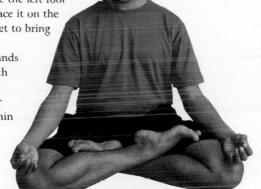

Repeat on the other side.

Need something easier?
If you have trouble with this posture you can always do a half lotus: raise one foot onto the opposite thigh and leave the other on the floor in a cross-legged position.

Trikonasana (THE TRIANGLE)

This posture gives a strong stretch on the legs. The sidebend helps to keep the back and the hips mobile.

1 Stand in *Tadasana* and step or jump the feet about 1 metre (3–4 feet) apart.
2 Raise your arms to shoulder height and stretch your fingers out, with your palms facing the floor.
3 Turn your right foot in slightly and your left foot out to the side, lining up your left heel with the arch of your right foot. Keep your hips, trunk and head facing forwards.
4 Breathe out and bend sideways to place your left hand on your left shin. Stretch the right arm up, with the palm facing forwards.
5 Check that your legs are straight and that your trunk and head are level with your legs and hips (they tend to lean forwards). Widen your upper chest and shoulders. Breathe gently and when you feel steady, look up towards your right hand.

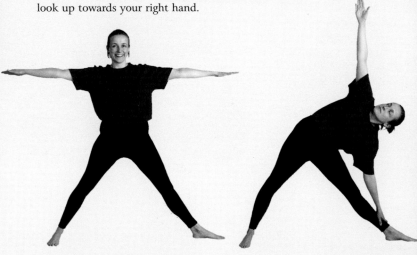

To come out, breathe in and lift your trunk up with your arms still stretching. Turn your feet forwards and repeat on the other side from step 3.

Parsvakonasana

This posture provides a good stretch for the legs, the hips and the sides of the trunk.

1 Stand in *Tadasana* and step or jump the feet about 1–1.5 metres (4–5 feet) apart.
2 Raise your arms to shoulder height and stretch your fingers out, with your palms facing the floor.
3 Turn your right foot in slightly and your left foot out to the side, lining up your left heel with the arch of your right foot. Keep your hips and trunk facing forwards.
4 Breathe out and bend your left knee to a right angle. Place the fingers of your left hand behind the left foot. (If your knee doesn't bend to a right angle, you may need to adjust your legs by taking them wider apart or closer together.)
5 Check that your right leg is straight. Open your chest and shoulders to face forwards. Raise your right arm and stretch it over your right ear, with your palm facing the floor.
6 Breathe gently and feel a strong stretch from your left foot through the side of your trunk to your right hand.

To come out, breathe in, straighten the right leg and bring your arms to the horizontal position. Turn both feet to the front and repeat on the other side from step 3.

Need something easier?
This is quite a tough posture if you are new to yoga. If necessary, place your outstretched hand on the back of a chair or against a wall for support.

Vrksasana (THE TREE)

This posture provides an excellent upward stretch. It requires a good sense of balance, however.

1 Stand in *Tadasana* and focus your eyes on a spot at eye level in front of you. Take hold of the right ankle with the right hand, bend the leg and place the heel of the foot on the inside of the left thigh.
2 When you feel steady, breathe out and stretch your arms upwards with your palms facing in.
3 Check that your standing leg is straight and that the left knee is turned to the side as far as possible.

To come out, breathe in and lower the arms to your sides. Lower the left leg and return to *Tadasana*. Repeat on the other side from step 1.

Need something easier?
Balancing takes some practise and if you're new to yoga you may find this one difficult. To give yourself more confidence, stand close to a wall so you can steady yourself if you start to overbalance.

Ardha chandrasana
(THE HALF MOON)

This is a fairly advanced balancing/standing posture which stretches the legs and opens the hips and shoulders.

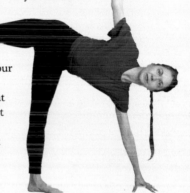

1   Stand in *Tadasana*, then go into *Trikonasana* on your left-hand side.
2   Lower your right arm and place your hand on your waist.
3   Bend your left knee to a right angle and place your left hand in a cupped position about 20–30cm (8–12 inches) from your left foot. Step your right foot in slightly.
4   Breathe out and straighten your left leg, at the same time lifting your right leg so that it comes to a horizontal position.
5   Check that your legs are straight and that your hips and trunk are facing forwards. If you feel steady, raise your right arm.

To come out, breathe in, lower your right leg to the floor and return to *Trikonasana*. Breathe in and lift your arms and trunk. Turn your feet to the front, lower your arms and repeat on the other side.

> ### Need something easier?
> This posture is not as daunting if you do it with your back to a wall. Position yourself about 20cm (8 inches) away from the wall so that you don't bump into it. You may also find this posture more comfortable if you place the fingers of your lower hand on a firm block.

Uttanasana

This basic standing forward bend is especially good for stretching the hamstrings.

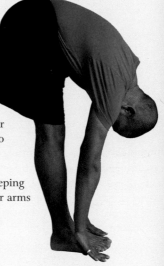

1 Stand in *Tadasana*, breathe in and raise your arms over your head, with your palms facing forwards. Stretch up tall.
2 Breathe out and lower your trunk and arms down, keeping your back concave for as long as possible. Place your fingers on the floor beside your feet and relax your neck and head down.
3 Stretch your legs, pushing up the tops of your thighs and draw the trunk down and closer to the legs as you breathe out.

To come out, breathe in and raise your trunk, keeping your back as straight as possible, and stretch your arms up over the head. Lower your arms.

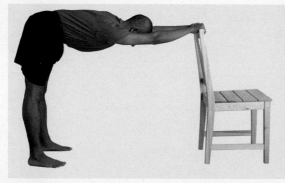

Need something easier?
A simpler version of this is the warm-up exercise Back 2 on page 12, where you stand with your legs hip-width apart and rest your hands on a support.

Pascimottonasana

This seated position stretches the hamstrings and the back muscles.

1 Sit on a block with your legs outstretched in front of you. Using your hands, part the flesh of your buttocks to the sides so that you are sitting on your 'buttock bones'.
2 Breathe out and lean forwards to take hold of your feet with both hands.
3 Check that your legs are straight and feel that you are leaning forwards from the hips and not from higher up the spine. The lower back should feel concave. Hold the shoulders wide so that the chest is open.
4 If you can bend lower, take the upper chest and head towards the shins. Clasp the hands round the feet, holding the wrist of one arm with the other hand.

To come out, breathe in, release the hands and lift the trunk, keeping the back straight.

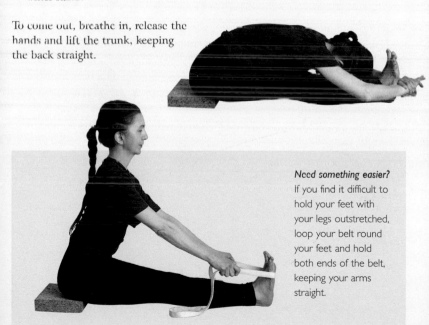

Need something easier?
If you find it difficult to hold your feet with your legs outstretched, loop your belt round your feet and hold both ends of the belt, keeping your arms straight.

25

Bhujangasana (THE COBRA)

This posture is a basic backbend which arches the back. If you have back problems you may need to avoid all backbends – consult your doctor to find out if this is the case.

1 Lie face down on the floor with your legs and feet together. Bend your elbows and place your hands on the floor at either side of your trunk about level with your chest, with your fingers apart and facing forwards.
2 Breathe in and straighten the arms so that the trunk lifts off the floor.
3 Check that your legs are straight, that your upper thighs are pushing down into the floor and that your chest and shoulders are open.
4 If you feel comfortable to do so, drop your head back and look upwards.

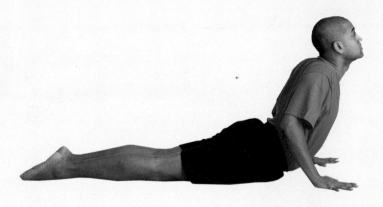

To come out, breathe out, bend the arms and lower the trunk to the floor.

Need something harder?
If you have a quite a flexible spine, place your hands on the floor closer to your waist. When you lift your trunk, make sure that you don't lift the tops of your thighs (your pubis bone) off the floor.

Ustrasana (THE CAMEL)

*This is quite a strong backbend which arches the back and opens out
the shoulders and upper chest. Avoid it if you have back problems or
consult your doctor about doing the easier version outlined at the
bottom of the page.*

1 Kneel up, with the knees and feet together
   and the trunk upright. Place the hands on
   the hips.
2 Holding the hips and the thighs in an
   upright position, breathe out and lean
   backwards to place the hands on the heels.
3 Check that your thighs and hips are not
   leaning backwards.
4 If you feel comfortable, drop your head back and
   look upwards.

To come out, breathe in and lift your trunk evenly
on both sides (make sure you push up from both
hands at the same time).

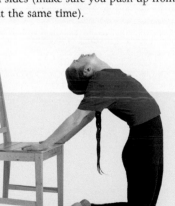

Need something easier?
If you find this too strong an arch
on your back, place a chair in front
of a wall and kneel down with your
back to it. Do the same as above
but when you lean back, place your
hands on the seat of the chair.
Drop your head backwards if it
feels comfortable.

27

Bharadjvasana

This simple twist can be excellent for a bad back – although for some back problems, twists are not advised (consult your doctor if this might be the case).

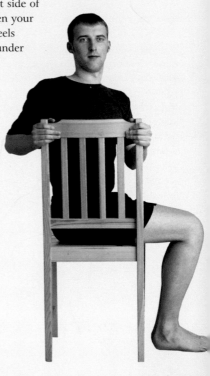

1 Sit sideways on a chair with the right side of the body against the chair back. Open your chest and shoulders wide. (If your heels don't touch the floor, place a block under your feet.)
2 Breathe out and turn your trunk towards the back of the chair, taking hold of the back of the chair.
3 With each out-breath, turn a little further round to the right. Make sure that your legs and knees stay in their original position.
4 Keeping your chest and shoulders open, turn your head and look over your right shoulder.

To come out, breathe in, release the hands and turn the trunk to face forwards. Stand up and sit on the other side of the chair with the left side of the body against the chair back. Repeat the twist on this side.

Parivrtta trikonasana
(REVERSE TRIANGLE)

This is a fairly advanced standing twist that requires a good sense of balance.

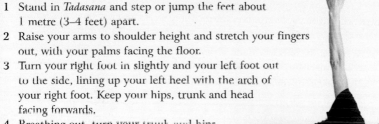

1 Stand in *Tadasana* and step or jump the feet about
   1 metre (3–4 feet) apart.
2 Raise your arms to shoulder height and stretch your fingers
   out, with your palms facing the floor.
3 Turn your right foot in slightly and your left foot out
   to the side, lining up your left heel with the arch of
   your right foot. Keep your hips, trunk and head
   facing forwards.
4 Breathing out, turn your trunk and hips
   as far round to the left as you can
   and place your right hand on your
   left shin. You should now be looking
   behind you.
5 Check your shoulders and
   chest are open, with the left
   shoulder above the right
   shoulder. Both legs should
   be straight and your
   left arm should be
   stretching upwards.

To come out, breathe in and lift the trunk and arms to face forwards.
Turn your feet to the front and repeat from step 3 on the other side.

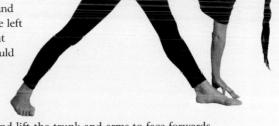

Need something easier?

If you feel unsteady, place a chair on the outside of your front foot and, rather than place
your hand on your shin, place your lower arm on the seat of the chair. This will give you
support to balance and should enable you to turn your chest a little more.

Sarvangasana (SHOULDER STAND) and Halasana (THE PLOUGH)

These are the most practised of the upside-down, or inverted, postures. They should not be practised during menstruation, nor if you suffer from high blood pressure.

1 Fold up three or four blankets so that you have a fairly high platform with a neat edge down one side for your neck to extend over.
2 Lie on your back with your trunk and shoulders on the platform, your head on the floor and the back of the neck long. Bend your knees and place your feet close to your buttocks.
3 Breathe out and lift the trunk, bending the legs over the head and supporting your upper back with your hands, the fingers spread wide.
4 Raise the trunk and stretch up the legs.
5 Check that your trunk and legs are vertical and above your shoulders and that your hands are firmly supporting your upper back. Do not attempt to move your head or neck, simply look towards your upper chest.

6 Lower your legs over your head and place your toes on the floor to come down into *Halasana*. Stretch your legs through to your heels and push your thighs up to the ceiling.

To come out, support your lower back with your hands and uncurl slowly. Do not sit up immediately, but find a comfortable resting position on the floor with the back of your neck extended.

Need something easier?

You may fear that you'll be unsteady in *Sarvangasana*, but using a chair in the following way will help you feel more confident:

1 Place a chair against a wall and lie on your back with your lower legs bent over the chair seat and your hands holding the front chair legs. (As before, your shoulders and upper back should be resting on the blanket platform.)
2 Breathing out, lift your bottom off the floor and place your feet on the edge of the chair seat. Breathe out again, raise your trunk and come up on to your shoulders, still holding the chair legs.
3 Stretch up through your spine and thighs and look at your chest with your eyes relaxed. (You may wish to lift your trunk and legs from here into a vertical position.)

To come out, lower your hips to the floor. Stay there a moment, relaxing the neck and then roll to the side.

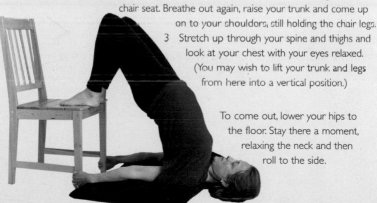

31

Relax

WITH

*M*ental stress and physical tension are two common problems that can be relieved by practising yoga. The stretching exercises and postures ease out tension in the muscles, while the concentration required to perform them helps many people unwind mentally.

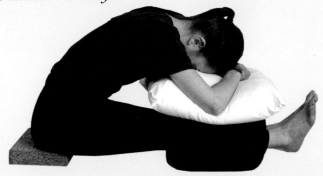

Yoga

While the relief of physical and mental stress is ongoing as you practise the postures, the most potent opportunity for relaxing comes at the end of a session. Having put in a lot of effort, you can now enjoy your 'reward' in the form of a relaxation period. The relaxation postures are used not only to release fully any tension that may remain in your muscles, but also to calm the mind. By focusing on something as simple as your breathing for just a short while, you can make the essential break from any anxieties that may be preoccupying you.

This section has several postures suitable for relaxation, as well as two basic relaxation techniques – deep breathing and the 'tense and let go' method. The exact time you spend in a relaxation posture is up to you, but aim for at least five minutes.

Savasana (THE CORPSE)

This is the most commonly used posture for relaxation. You will need a blanket.

1 Lie down on the floor with your head supported on a folded blanket.
2 Move the shoulders away from the head and flatten the shoulder blades into the back. Feel that the chest is wide and open.
3 Relax the abdomen and the lower back so that the space beneath your lower back is reduced.
4 Extend the arms and hands away from the body, placing them on the floor with the palms facing upwards and the fingers gently curled.
5 Extend the legs and feet and let them fall apart, with the toes pointing slightly outwards.
6 Stretch out the back of the neck so that the back of the skull rests on the support. Feel that your forehead is smooth and your mouth is relaxed.
7 Close your eyes and quieten your breathing so that it's even and rhythmic.

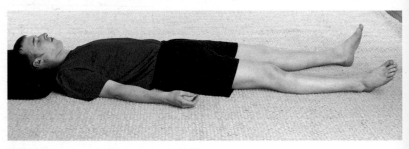

To come out, open your eyes and slowly turn onto one side.
Remain there for 30 seconds or so before sitting up.

Need something for your lower back?
If your lower back feels uncomfortable in this position, place a firm cushion under your knees and lower legs to raise them slightly. To get a higher angle, lift up your lower legs and place them on the seat of a chair.

Pascimottonasana

This is the relaxed version of the forward bend shown on page 25.
You will need a few blankets or cushions.

1   Sit on a block with your legs outstretched in front of you. Place your
    blankets or cushions in a pile over your shins (fold the blankets carefully so
    that they are flat).
2   Bend forwards and place your forehead on the support. Stretch your arms
    forwards to rest over the support.
3   Relax the spine and try not to move the head from side to side.

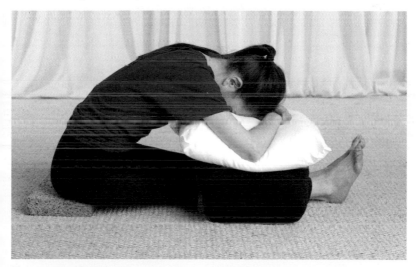

To come out, breathe in and slowly uncurl the spine.

Need something higher?
If you don't feel entirely comfortable with your support, position a chair over your legs
with a blanket or cushion on the seat and rest your chin on it, with your arms folded on
the chair seat.

35

Supta baddha konasana
(THE COBBLER)

This is the relaxed version of the Cobbler. You will need your belt, as well as a few blankets and a block.

1   Make a platform for your back out of blankets. Fold them so they are long enough to extend from the base of your spine to beyond your head. Place the block at the far end to support your head.
2   Sit on the floor in front of your support, with your knees bent out to the sides and the soles of your feet touching.
3   Take your belt and pass one end behind the waist, over your thighs and round your feet. Buckle it to the other end so that it is quite tight and the buckle lies over your shins but not against your skin.
4   Check that you are lined up with your support and, breathing out, lower your back onto the support. Position the block under your head.
5   Fold your arms behind your head or place them on the floor at your sides.

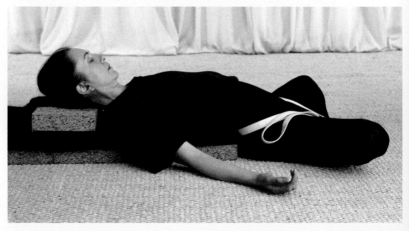

To come out, push up on your hands from the floor and sit up. Remove the belt.

Setubandha sarvangasana

This relaxing posture is a slight backbend. You should never finish a session with a backbend, so always do another relaxation posture after this one. You will need a few blankets or firm cushions.

1 Make a platform with your blankets or cushions, making sure they are flat.
2 Sit on the platform and lie back, placing your head and upper back on the floor behind you. Roll backwards slightly on your platform so that it is positioned just below the back of your waist.
3 Relax your legs, holding them quite close together. Fold your arms over your head.

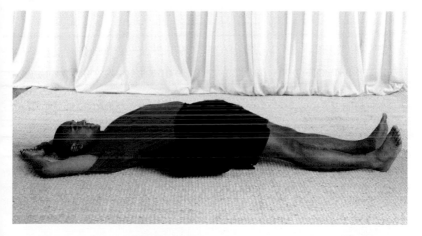

To come out, push your platform to the side, lower your bottom to the floor and sit up.

Need something to ease your lower back?
If your lower back is uncomfortable in this position, place a block under your feet so that your legs are raised to the same height as the platform.

Viparita karani

This is a very restful inverted posture. You will need some blankets or firm cushions.

1 Make a platform with your blankets or cushions and place it up against a wall. (The cushions should be firm or you'll slip off them.)
2 Sit sideways on your platform with one hip touching the wall and your feet and hands on the floor.
3 Swing your legs up and place them against the wall, then lower your back to the floor.
4 Check that your bottom is very close in to the wall. If it isn't, shuffle it further on to the platform.
5 Relax your back and shoulders and fold your arms over your head. Hold your legs close together.
6 If you wish, you can bend your knees to either side and bring the soles of your feet together.

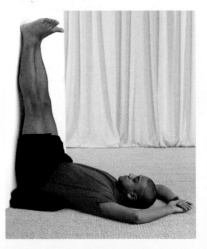
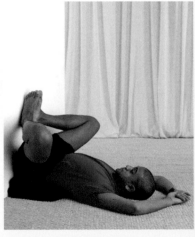

To come out, bend your knees and, with your feet against the wall, push your bottom off the platform on to the floor. Roll over to one side and sit up.

Relaxation exercises

DEEP BREATHING

Breathing a little more deeply than usual can be a very relaxing experience. It settles and concentrates the mind.

1 Choose one of the relaxation postures and check that you are totally comfortable and not likely to feel restless.
2 Breathe normally for a minute or so through your nostrils, listening to the sound of your breath and feeling your chest rise and fall.
3 Begin your deep breathing by breathing out for slightly longer than usual.
4 Breathe in slowly and deeply, feeling your rib cage expand.
5 If this feels comfortable, continue with an equally long out-breath and then regular in- and out-breaths of more or less equal length. Feel that your breathing extends into your abdomen as your diaphragm moves up and down.
6 Return to shorter more shallow breathing before coming up.

If you felt any tension in your face, neck or chest you may have been trying to breathe too slowly and deeply, exerting too much pressure on your lungs.

TENSE AND LET GO

This relaxation method releases any tension that may be left in your body after your practice session. It involves working through your body – from head to toe or toe to head – tensing and then relaxing the muscles until you are completely relaxed. The method is simple, although it may take a few practices to perfect.

1 Choose one of the relaxation postures and check that you are totally comfortable and not likely to feel restless.
2 One by one, starting at the head or toes, tense each muscle group – curl your toes, make a fist of your hands, tighten your stomach muscles, hunch your shoulders, screw up your face, etc. – and then, once you are sure it could not be any more tense, let it go completely. Keep your breathing smooth as you work through the body.
3 When you have relaxed the whole body, breathe in and out evenly – and enjoy the restfulness and calm.

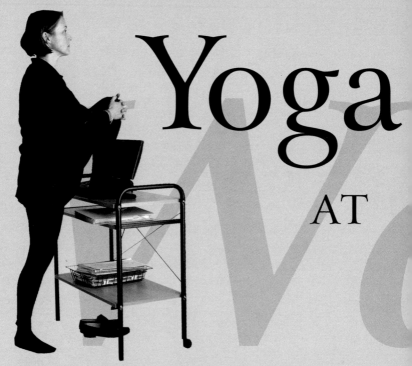

Yoga

AT

F ortunately, yoga is a form of exercise that can be practised almost anywhere. If you suffer from job-related stress, you might benefit greatly from taking a few minutes out to stretch and relax while you are at work.

In this section you will find references to some exercises and postures that are described in earlier sections, as well as some new ones that are suited to a work environment. Many of the exercises can be performed discreetly at your desk, others require some space and a wall that you can lean against.

Work

A short sequence of exercises and postures is also featured. This is designed to stretch your muscles and joints gently and quieten and relax the body and mind, and can be carried out when you have about ten minutes spare.

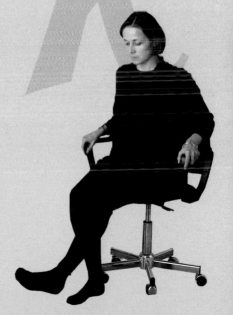

Seated postures

For this set of exercises and postures all you need is a chair in which you can sit up straight and still place your feet on the floor. (If your chair seat is too high, place a book or two under your feet.) These exercises and the posture can be practised as a sequence or just one or two at a time.

NECK

The warm-up exercise Neck 1 (see page 9) is suited to a work environment.

SHOULDERS

Both warm-up exercises Shoulders 1 and 2 (see page 10) can be practised while you are seated (below).

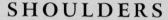

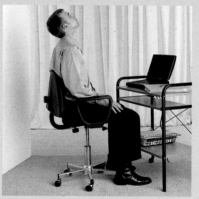

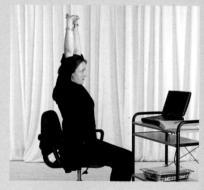

WRISTS

The first warm-up exercise for your wrists Wrists 1 (see page 11) can be practised while sitting. Sit forward on your chair so that you have enough space behind your back to position your hands.

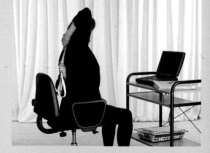

BACK

The yoga posture *Bharadjvasana* (see page 28) can be practised on your chair. Ensure that you can place your feet together, flat on the floor.

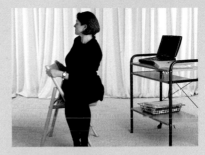

KNEES & FEET

This exercise stretches the muscles of your knees and feet. You can practise it discreetly at your desk but ideally you will need to take off your shoes.

1 Sitting with your back erect, stretch your legs out in front of you and point your toes. Breathe gently as you curl your toes.
2 Relax the feet and then push the heels away from you as you pull the toes towards you.
3 Breathe gently and feel a strong stretch behind the knees.
4 Relax the feet and repeat.

ANKLES

This is another discreet exercise that you can practise under your desk. It is best if you can take off your shoes.

1 With your knees bent and your feet placed on the floor, lift up your right foot and rotate it in one direction a couple of times.
2 Stop and rotate it in the other direction a couple of times.
3 Repeat with the other foot.
4 Go back to the first foot and try to make the rotation wider each time.
5 Repeat with the other foot.

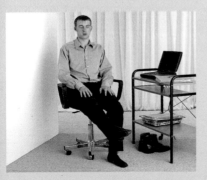

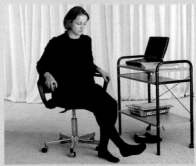

Standing postures

For this set of exercises you just need some space, a surface such as a desk or a windowsill, and a wall. These exercises can be practised as a sequence or just one or two at a time.

SHOULDERS

This exercise can give quite a strong stretch to the shoulder muscles. You will need a wall.

1 Stand at right angles to the wall with your right foot about 10cm (4 inches) away from it.
2 Lift your right arm and place your hand against the wall, level with your shoulder.
3 Keeping the shoulder close in to the wall, breathe out and gently turn your chest away from the wall.
4 Breathe gently and, with each out-breath, turn the chest into the room.
5 Relax your arm, turn round and repeat with the other arm and shoulder.

BACK

Both warm-up exercises Back 1 and 2 (see page 12) are suited to a work environment and work clothes, if they are loose enough. You will need to take off your shoes unless they are flat.

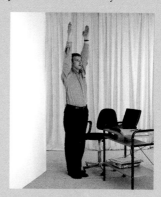

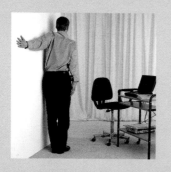

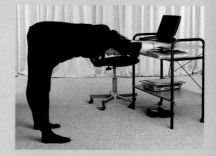

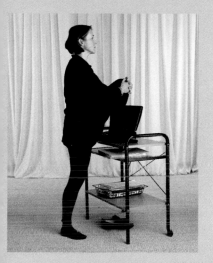
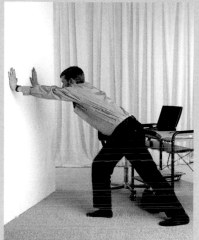

HIPS

This exercise can only be practised if
you are wearing loose-fitting trousers.
You will need to find a ledge which is
comfortable to place your foot upon –
this could be a desk, a windowsill or a
low bookcase. You will need to take
off your shoes.

1 Stand tall and face the ledge.
2 Lift your left leg and place your
   foot on the ledge, with your left
   knee pointing up to the ceiling.
3 Fold your arms over your knee and
   look ahead.
4 Check that your right leg is
   straight and that your left hip is
   not tilted outwards. (Find a lower
   surface if this is the case.)
5 Lower your left leg and repeat on
   the other side.

KNEES & ANKLES

This is an excellent exercise for
stretching out the back of your knees,
calves and ankles. You will need a wall.

1 Stand facing the wall at a distance
   of about half a metre (2 feet).
2 Step your right foot towards the
   wall and place your hands on the
   wall. Your right knee should be
   bent and your left leg straight.
3 Breathe out as you push your left
   heel down into the floor. If this
   feels too easy, step your left foot
   back slightly or bend your right
   knee a little lower. You should feel
   the stretch at the back of the left
   knee and down into the calf.
4 Step your right leg back, stand
   up straight and repeat on the
   other side.

A short sequence

This short sequence of exercises followed by a few moments of quiet relaxation can be carried out in a minimum of about ten minutes. You will need a wall, a surface to lean on and a chair – and no interruptions, if possible!

1 Standing, start with warm-up exercise Neck 1 (see page 9).

3 Still standing, move on to the shoulders exercise shown on page 44.

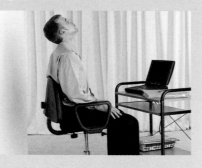

2 Move on to warm-up exercise Back 1 (see page 12).

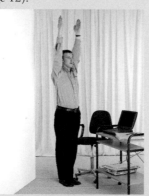

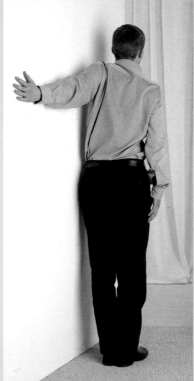

4 Find a surface to place your hands on and do warm-up exercise Back 2 (see page 12).

5 Find a wall and do the knees and ankles exercise shown on page 45.

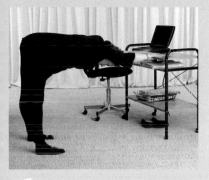

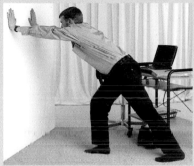

6 Sit down on your chair and do the ankles exercise described on page 43.

7 Do the exercise Wrists 1 (see page 11).

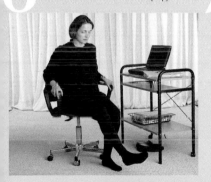

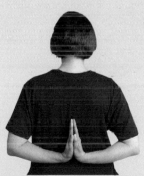

8 Place your hands in your lap, sit erect, close your eyes and start to quieten down your breathing. When you feel ready, practise either of the Relaxation exercises (see page 39).

Return your breathing to normal, open your eyes and take in your surroundings. You should now feel refreshed and ready to start work again!

Yoga

AND

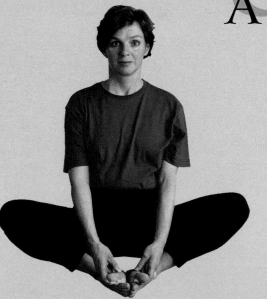

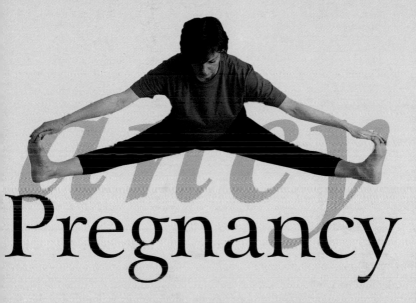

Pregnancy

If ever a woman needed to maintain her body in the best possible shape, it is during pregnancy.

Yoga is recommended for this purpose for the following reasons:

- it helps create a feeling of physical well-being and can relieve tension
- it strengthens muscles and mobilizes joints
- it helps the body adapt to the increasing weight and alteration in balance
- it improves lung function, giving a better oxygen supply to both mother and baby

General advice during and after pregnancy

If you haven't practised yoga before and are considering taking it up for the first time when you are pregnant, it is recommended that you attend an ante-natal yoga class to receive expert guidance from a teacher. This book can then be used as a companion guide.

For those women who have been practising yoga for some time and have a certain level of yoga knowledge and body awareness, many of the exercises and postures described earlier in this book and in this section can be practised in the home – as long as you don't overstretch, and you feel comfortable at all times. Note that some yoga teachers suggest that you shouldn't attempt any backbends or twists at all during pregnancy.

The postures in this section are designed to strengthen your back and stretch the muscles in the pelvic floor area in the months leading up to the birth. They can be practised as far into your pregnancy as possible.

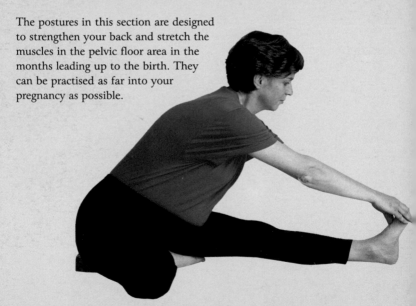

Baddha konasana
(THE COBBLER)

This posture can prepare the pelvic floor by stretching and toning the muscles in that area. The upward stretch on the back helps to keep the back strong. You will need a block or blanket.

1 Sit on a block or a folded blanket with your legs outstretched in front of you.
2 Bend your legs, dropping your knees to the sides and draw the feet up close to the body with the soles touching.
3 Hold the feet with both hands.
4 Check that you are sitting upright and that your lower back is not arched. With each out-breath feel that you are opening up the pelvic area and gently easing the knees towards the floor.

To come out, release the hands and straighten the legs.

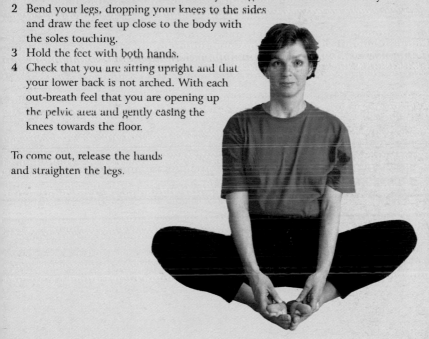

Need something more restful?
If you find this posture tiring, sit with your back against a wall. Using your hand, check that your lower back is not arched.

Malasana

This is a modification of a fairly advanced posture, making it much more manageable. It is excellent for opening up the pelvic area and strengthening the back. You will need a blanket and a chair.

1 Roll up your blanket and place it on the floor about 30 cm (1 foot) in front of the chair.
2 Stand, facing the chair, with the heels of your feet on the edge of the blanket and the balls of your feet on the floor.
3 Bending at the hips, squat down to take hold of the chair seat with both hands.
4 Breathe smoothly, press your heels down into the blanket and keep your back straight. This is a good opportunity to practise your pelvic floor exercises.

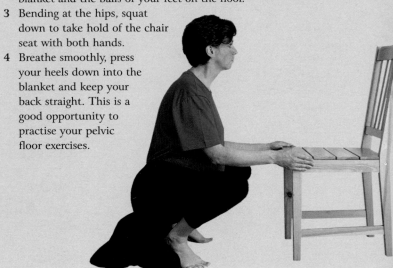

To come out, place more of your weight on the chair seat, and use it as a support as you straighten your legs and stand up.

Need something harder?
If you have quite flexible ankles, try this posture with your heels on the floor rather than on the blanket.

Janu sirsasana

This is a sitting forward bend that you should be able to practise quite far into your pregnancy. You will need a block and possibly your belt.

1 Sit on a block with your legs outstretched in front of you. Using your hands, part the flesh of your buttocks to the sides so that you are sitting on your 'buttock bones'.
2 Bend your right leg and bring the right knee down to the side so that it is close to the floor. Place the sole of your right foot against or slightly under your left thigh.
3 Sit up tall, breathe out and lean forwards to take hold of your left foot with both hands. (If you cannot reach easily, take your belt, hold it in both hands and hook it round your foot.)
4 Check that your left leg is straight and that you are leaning forwards from the hips. Hold the shoulders wide so that the chest is open.

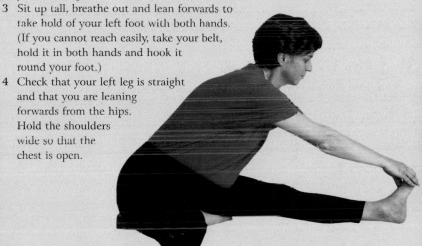

To come out, breathe in, release your hands (or belt) and lift the trunk, keeping the back straight. Repeat on the other side

Need something more restful?

If you prefer something more relaxing, place some folded blankets or cushions over your shins and rest your head on them.

53

Upavista konasana

This posture gives the pelvic area and thighs an excellent stretch, but be careful that you don't overstretch the inside thigh muscles. You will need a block.

1 Sit on a block with your legs outstretched in front of you. Use your hands to part the flesh of your buttocks to the sides so that you are sitting on your 'buttock bones'.
2 Keeping your back straight, take your legs apart, with the knees and toes facing upwards. (Don't take your legs too far apart – keep them within your 'comfort' limit.)
3 Sit up tall, breathe out and lean forwards to take hold of each foot with the corresponding hand. (If you cannot reach easily, place your hands on your shins, or if you have two belts hook one round each foot.)
4 Check that both legs are straight and that you are leaning forwards from the hips. With each out-breath see if you can lower yourself slightly further down (but don't overstretch).

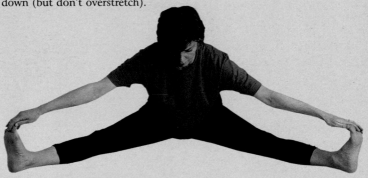

To come out, breathe in, release your hands and straighten your back.

Need something more restful?
If you prefer something more relaxing, place a chair or a pile of folded blankets on the floor in front of you and rest your head on them.

Adho mukha svanasana
(THE DOG)

This is a restful variation of the warm-up exercise Knees 1 (see page 14). It is a good all-round stretch which also rests the heart. You will need a block or folded blanket.

1 Kneel on the floor and place your folded blanket or block in front of you. Place your hands, shoulder-width apart, just in front of the blanket. Spread your fingers wide apart.
2 Lift your knees off the floor and check that your feet are level and about hip-width apart.
3 Breathing out, straighten your legs and lift the hips up high. Your weight should be balanced between your toes and balls of the feet and your hands.
4 Breathe out again and lower your heels towards the floor (if they touch easily step your feet back). You will feel a stretch in your hamstrings and calf muscles.
5 Place your forehead on your support.
6 You should feel a strong stretch through your arms, trunk and down your legs while your face and head remain relaxed.

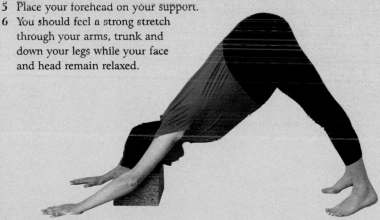

To come out, bend the knees and kneel with your knees apart. Rest your trunk forwards in a comfortable position, place your forearms on the support and rest your head down for a few moments before coming up.

Yoga

*T*his section features three programmes for yoga practice,
each one made up of warm-up exercises and postures
described earlier. If an exercise or posture doesn't suit you,
replace it with something similar that you like, or leave it out.
These programmes are quite flexible, so adapt them, if necessary,
to find something that you enjoy doing and will look forward to.

The first programme, a morning energizer, is designed to wake you up,
stretch muscles, loosen joints and so set you up for the day. In the
second programme, an evening energizer, the postures are more hard-
working and include a backbend and an inverted posture.

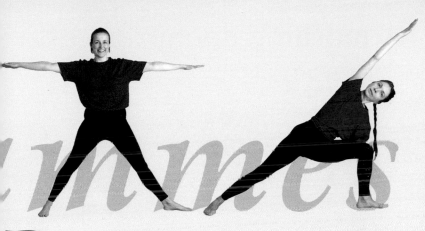

Programmes

Neither of these programmes have to be practised at these times of day. You can do them whenever you feel like it. The third programme is a sequence of relaxation postures suitable for any occasion.

The duration of each programme is not given but assume that you will need a minimum of 20 minutes – and more for the third programme to be really effective.

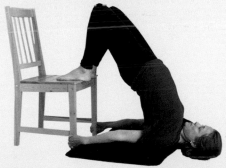

A morning energizer

You will need your belt, a chair and a blanket or cushion.

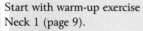

1 Start with warm-up exercise Neck 1 (page 9).

4 Take your belt and do warm-up exercise Hips 1 (page 13).

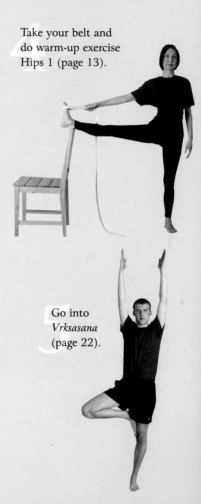

2 Move on to warm-up exercise Back 1 (page 12).

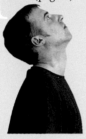

5 Go into *Vrksasana* (page 22).

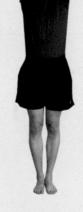

3 Now do warm-up exercise Shoulders 1 (page 10).

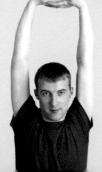

Come back into *Tadasana* (page 18) and then go into *Trikonasana* (page 20).

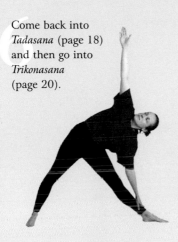

Come back into *Tadasana* and then go into *Parsvakonasana* (page 21).

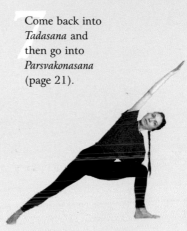

Come back into *Tadasana* and then go into *Uttanasana* (page 24).

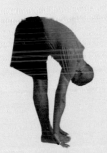

Sit sideways on a chair and do *Bharadjvasana* (page 28).

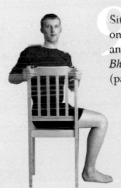

Finish off by relaxing in *Savasana* (page 34) with a blanket or cushion under your head.

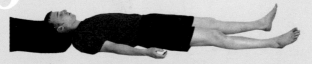

An evening energizer

You will need your belt, blankets and a block.

1 Start with warm-up exercise Feet and ankles 1 (page 15).

2 Take your belt and move on to warm-up exercise Knees 2 (page 14).

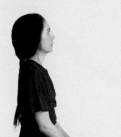

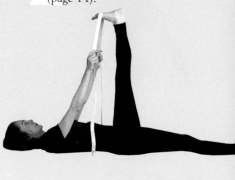

3 Now do warm-up exercise Hips 2 (page 13).

4 Now move on to do warm-up exercise Back 2 (page 12).

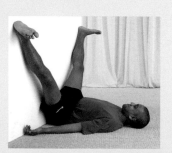

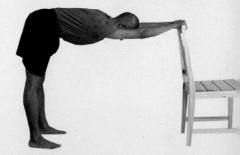

Using the belt, if necessary, do warm-up exercise Shoulders 2 (page 10).

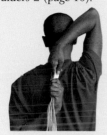

Then move into *Ustrasana* (page 27).

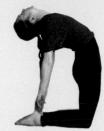

Now do warm-up exercise Knees 1 (page 14).

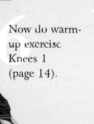

Sit sideways on a chair and do *Bharadjvasana* (page 28).

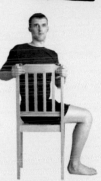

Lie on the floor and do *Bhujangasana* (page 26).

Take up your blankets and do *Sarvangasana* and *Halasana* (pages 30–1).

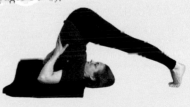

Relax in *Savasana* (page 34) with a blanket or cushion under your head.

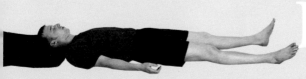

Relaxation

You will need your belt, blankets and one or more blocks.

1 Take up your blankets and start with *Viparita karani* (page 38).

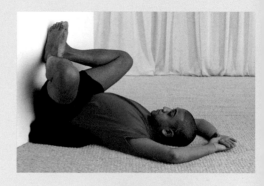

2 Move on to *Adho mukha svanasana* (page 14) with a block under your head.

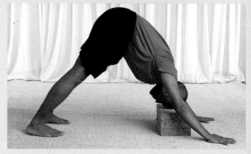

3 Reposition your blankets and blocks and do *Supta baddha konasana* (page 36), with your belt round your legs.

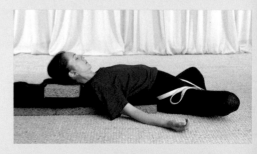

Remake your blankets
or use blocks and do
Setubandha sarvangasana
(page 37).

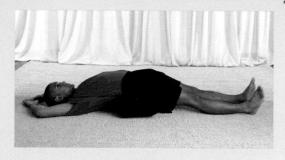

Sit on a block and use a pile of
blankets on your shins for *Janu
sirsasana* (page 53).

Stay with block and blankets and do
Pascimottonasana (page 35).

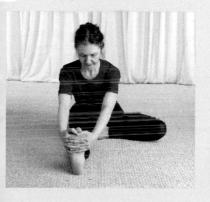

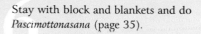
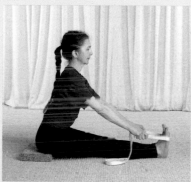

Finish off with *Savasana* (page 34) with a blanket or cushion under your head.

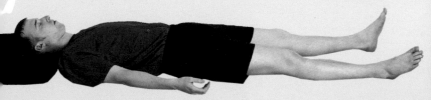

Index

Adho mukha svanasana, 55
aids, 6
ankles
    warm-up exercises, 15
    yoga at work, 43, 44
Ardha chandrasana, 23
arms see shoulders; wrists

back
    Bharadjvasana, 28
    Bhujangasana, 26
    Pascimottonasana, 25
    Setubandha
        sarvangasana, 37
    Ustrasana, 27
    warm-up exercises, 12
    yoga at work, 43, 44
Baddha konasana, 51
balance
    Ardha chandrasana, 23
    Vrksasana, 22
Bharadjvasana, 28
Bhujangasana, 26
breathing exercises, 39

Camel, The, 27
Cobbler, The, 36, 51
Cobra, The, 26
Corpse, The, 34

Dog, The, 55

evening energizer
    programme, 60–1

feet
    warm-up exercises, 15
    yoga at work, 43
forward bends
    Pascimottonasana, 25, 34
    Uttanasana, 24

Halasana, 30–1
Half Moon, The, 23
hamstrings,
Pascimottonasana, 25
hips
    Parsvakonasana, 21
    warm-up exercises, 13
    yoga at work, 44

inverted postures
    Halasana, 30–1
    Sarvangasana, 30–1
    Viparita karani, 38

Janu sirsasana, 53

knees
    warm-up exercises, 14
    yoga at work, 43, 44

legs
    Parsvakonasana, 21
    Pascimottonasana, 25
    Trikonasana, 20
    see also ankles; feet;
    hips; knees
Lotus, The, 19

Malasana, 52
meditation, Lotus position, 19
morning energizer
    programme, 58–9
Mountain, The, 18

neck
    warm-up exercises, 9
    yoga at work, 42

Padmasana, 19
Parivrtta trikonasana, 29
Parsvakonasana, 21
Pascimottonasana, 25, 35

pelvic floor muscles, 51
Plough, The, 30–1
pregnancy, 48–55
relaxation, 32–9, 62–3
Reverse Triangle, 29

Sarvangasana, 30–1
Savasana, 34
seated postures, yoga at
    work, 42–3
Setubandha sarvangasana, 37
shoulders
    Shoulder Stand, 30–1
    warm-up exercises, 10
    yoga at work, 42, 44
standing postures, yoga at
    work, 44–5
stretching exercises, 16–31
Supta baddha konasana, 36

Tadasana, 18
tense and let go exercise, 39
Tree, The, 22
Triangle, The, 20
    Reverse Triangle, 29
Trikonasana, 20
twists
    Bharadjvasana, 28
    Parivrtta trikonasana, 29

Upavista konasana, 54
Ustrasana, 27
Uttanasana, 24

Viparita karani, 38
Vrksasana, 22

warm-up exercises, 8–15
work, yoga at, 40–7
wrists
    warm-up exercises, 11
    yoga at work, 42